The Friendly Handbook of Knee Surgery Recovery for Women

Women Talk to Women about Coping Tips and Tricks after Knee Surgery

by

Bruce H. Wolk

First Printing, 2020

ISBN978-1719086738

Bruce H. Wolk

Made Here Books, LLC

Denver, Colorado 80220

CONTENTS

One Small Step at a Time

Does it seem that more women than ever are having some type of knee surgery? It's not your imagination. Of the nearly 700,000 knee replacements performed each year in the United States, about 64% of those replacements are done on women. The numbers keep rising. Of course, implants are only one knee surgery procedure. Arthroscopic surgery, for example, accounts for roughly 750,000 surgeries per year.

According to the Mayo Clinic, about 3 million women are currently living with a knee implant, as compared to 1.7 million men. Why the difference? The Centers for Disease Control and Prevention notes that arthritis is often to blame. About 26 percent of women are diagnosed with arthritis as compared to about 19 percent of men.

The average age at which women are getting knee replacements is *declining*. Between 2000 and 2010, the average age for knee replacements went from 69 years to 66 years, and why not? We want to live active lives for as long as possible. Anecdotally, several of the women we interviewed mentioned they were athletes in high school, college and beyond. They sustained knee injuries in team sports, at the gym or just rough-housing with the kids. The point is that knee surgery is not just an older woman's option.

Attitudes are changing. Back in 2008, *The New York Times* reported that women often delayed knee surgery until they could no longer stand the pain. While it is understandable that younger women especially might want to delay surgery until their children are older and more self-sufficient, their orthopedic surgeons would undoubtedly tell them same thing I heard when facing surgery: *there are no medals given out for living with pain.* Sooner or later the prospect of knee surgery may become a reality for you.

Your surgeon and her (or his) team are the experts on everything medical. Knee surgery and rehabilitation, from a minor procedure to a total replacement, has come a long way. Don't be afraid to talk things out and to discuss your options.

This book makes no attempt to tell you what to do in a surgical sense. All medical decisions must be between you and your healthcare provider.

However, if you decide to proceed, this book might add to your safety and comfort as you get back to your old fighting self.

The Scope of This Book

The Friendly Handbook of Knee Surgery Coping Tips and Tricks is based on first-person interviews, email and snail mail correspondence, stories and the observations of women knee surgery patients.

The Friendly Handbook of Knee Surgery Coping Tips and Tricks for Women gives practical advice as to how women coped with knee surgeries in the first few days, weeks and months after their procedures. As you read through the comments, the hope is that you will come away with some good ideas. We don't expect that all of the experiences will apply to everyone, though more than a few men have also found the tricks in this book to be of use, including me.

We need to again stress that this book is **NON-MEDICAL**. It *does not discuss* pain-killing or anti-inflammatory medications, medical symptoms or post-surgical problems. There are many online sources, books and pamphlets explaining knee surgery.

You are strongly urged to contact your medical provider about any medical concerns.

A warning about the social media knee surgery support groups: The groups are mostly helpful, but you might run into a "know-it-all" who has never seen the inside of a medical or nursing school.

Please steer clear of anyone who dispenses medical, surgical or pharmaceutical advice on a social media website. If you are in pain or you are having a reaction of any kind, immediately call your healthcare provider.

The Knee Surgery Patients

In all, 22 former patients were interviewed for *Knee Surgery Coping Tips and Tricks*. The book is arranged so that you can imagine the patients responding to the questions as though they are sitting around a large virtual community table.

The women are from all over North America. Everyone's name has been changed to maintain complete confidentiality. Although every woman responded to every question, in some cases, they gave nearly identical answers (so we picked the most creative or informative). In some cases, we picked the funniest as well!

Throughout the book are "Common Comments," that is, common points on which many of the participants agreed.

We know what some of you reading the comments might say: "Well, everyone knows that!" The comical part is that several women who commented said, "I thought I knew that too, but after surgery, I forgot!" It's easy to forget what you should do after surgery because you are unfocused.

The Women's Knee Recovery Group – "The Virtual Community Table"

The women who were kind enough to contribute their comments asked for anonymity. To the best of their knowledge, they described the procedures that their surgeons performed. Something that became clear was that "age" did not indicate how they coped. For example, 30-year-old Whitney learned to cope after surgery in much the same way as women twice her age. In other cases, an older woman (with the same surgery) may have had an easier time of recovery than someone much younger. What was clear, though, was that everyone wanted to help.

The Virtual Community Table

Name	Age	Procedure
Whitney	30	Arthroscopy with Lateral Release
Kayla	33	ACL Repair, Bone Spurs, Chondroplasty, Nerve Severing
Anne	35	Total Knee Replacements
Emilie	38	Arthroscopy
Jessica	42	Partial Knee Replacement, both knees previously scoped
Katherine	45	Total Knee Replacement
Jane	47	Total Knee Replacement
Babs	50	Total Knee Replacement
Pamela	51	Total Knee Replacement
Meredith	55	ACL Reconstruction with 2 bucket meniscus tears
Emma	56	Torn Meniscus Surgery
Tess	56	Partial Knee Replacements
Lori	57	ACL Reconstruction
Michelle	62	Total Knee Replacement
Suzie Q	65	Total Knee Replacements
Heather	67	Total Knee Replacements
Susan	67	Total Knee Replacements
Violet	68	Total Knee Replacement
Harriet	69	Arthroscopy, Injections
Sarah	71	Total Knee Replacement
Ruthie	71	Total Knee Replacement
Samantha	72	Total Knee Replacement

Common Comments: Happy Thoughts Right After Surgery

Question: *Immediately following surgery what is the advice you most remembered that others who went through surgery gave to you?*

1. This is your time to relax and heal. You've earned it.
2. You will be groggy for a few days so don't plan on doing much more than sleeping.
3. Let your friends entertain you! Rest and relax and let *them* bring *you* the chocolate chip cookies!
4. Don't be afraid to say, "I'm tired and I need my rest!"
5. Listen to your physical therapist or orthopedic surgeon. *Don't do more than they want you to do.*
6. On the other hand, *do what they want you to do* unless there is a problem. If there is, tell them!
7. It may not feel like your knee at first! You will get used to it until it's part of you.
8. *Immediately report problems* to your surgeon's office. They want to help.
9. If you have young children or pets get *assistance.* Kids may understand mommy is in pain, a large puppy won't!
10. Stay off of airplanes until your orthopedic surgeon tells you it is OK to fly.
11. Do *not drive* until your orthopedic surgeon or physical therapist says it's alright to do so.
12. Do as much as you can *from a safe position* such as sitting or lying in an elevated position.
13. If you feel the least bit unsteady, *please let someone help you!* It's OK to be a baby.
14. Do not be a hero. Repeat. Do not be a hero.
15. Tell your husband to cook his own damn dinner! (LOL)

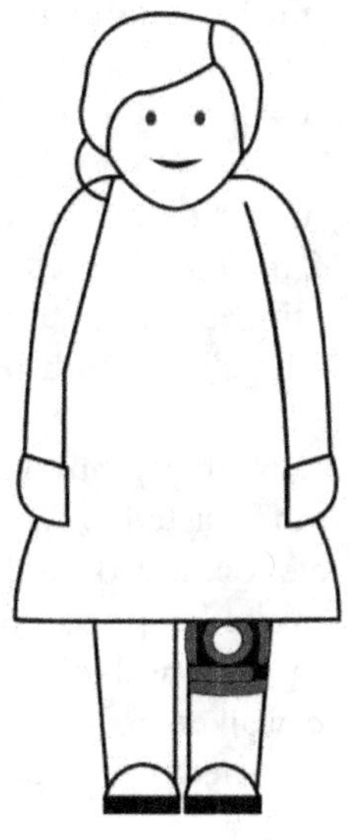

Chapter One: Moving About

Question: *How did you first get around after surgery, and as you got better what did you graduate to?*

[Note: Do not compare yourself to anybody else. Go at your own pace and listen to your orthopedic surgeon and physical therapist.]

"I thought I would be tougher, I guess. I started slowly with a walker and then I went to crutches. Looking back, my arms hurt very badly due to the crutches. I don't think I used them correctly. So, I want to say don't move to crutches too quickly! Stick with a walker or scooter for longer. I also struggled with balance. Allow yourself time to heal." Katherine

"I played volleyball in middle school, clubs, high school, and it got me a 4-yearcollegiate scholarship. I sacrificed my body. I am still young, I played sports, I thought I had all the upper body strength I needed. I thought I was hot stuff! After surgery I needed a walker to get around for several weeks, then I could use a cane. If I had to take my time, you will need to also." Anne

"I used a scooter most of the time, then I went to a walker and then a cane. I am too old for crutches. My balance was very off at first. I had a hard time getting around, but eventually I got the hang of it. My pain was not too bad." Samantha

"I was up with the help of my physical therapist three hours after leaving surgery for an assisted walk using the walker and he placed a 'gait belt' on me for added support. I walked 100 feet. When I was released from the hospital, I used a walker for a week and then transitioned to a quad walker. My first post-op visits to my surgeon, he took the walker away with instructions to use it only if I got dizzy from pain meds." Pamela

"I was first on crutches and then I got to slowly walking around without any crutches and sometimes a cane." Emma

"My procedure was no big deal compared to what others go through, but I was unsteady at first because I have a balance problem. Do not be a big shot. Do not attempt anything alone. Ask for help you're not Superwoman." Harriet

"I used a walker for a while then I graduated to a cane. It's going to take time. Listen to your physical therapist." Babs

"I used a walker and then I graduated to crutches after a little while." Sarah

"I was very weak after my surgery so I used a wheelchair for a while. I also have back issues which did not help. I feel like my back was aggravated after the knee surgery for some reason. After about 2 weeks I started using crutches." Lori

"At first I was on crutches and then I went to one crutch and then limping!" Kayla

"Because I did both knees at once, I used a walker and I needed it for a solid 8 weeks because neither leg was strong enough to hold me up! I graduated to a cane." Tess

"I recovered pretty quickly. I used a crutch and then a cane. I was never in any real pain." Emilie

"For the scope procedures I used crutches and after the replacement I used a walker for about a week to stabilize myself. I graduated to walking with assistance but cautiously. My biggest challenge was balance. My knee wanted to give out so I was very guarded. Take your time!" Jessica

Question: *Did you learn any tricks or tips about moving around those first days?*

"We quickly modified my walker by sticking 'furniture-foot' felts, to the rear legs of the walker. These are the kind with adhesive on one side. It was initially too much for me to push it [the walker] because I wasn't able to keep my balance. It was much easier to push the walker and have it slide on our wood floors. We went through many packages of these [felts] once I started walking outside!" Tess

"We have wooden floors too! My slippers were too slippery (duh!) but I am so glad I brought home two pairs of those hospital socks with the rubber grips on the bottom. It's always good to be friendly to the nurses!" Emilie

"I did not know what to expect. Before surgery I took up all of the slippery area rugs and made sure there were no electrical cords on the floor. If you have pets or kids make sure they leave no toys around where you're sitting." Harriet

"Buy a pair of pajama bottoms made of a slippery fabric such as nylon. It was so much easier than sweat pants to scoot myself to the edge of the bed and to slide up from a reclining position to a sitting position on the bed." Michelle

"I had two walkers – one for my main level and one for the upstairs bedroom. Before I could climb stairs, I used two of them on the main level. A suggestion I got from a co-worker who had foot surgery was to look in thrift stores for lightly used walkers. There's plenty. You can pick one or more up for a reasonable price (under $20). It also works to have more walkers on one level if you have a home with narrow doorways." Susie Q

"I went through this twice. I already knew after the first time that moving around could be dangerous. I cleared all throw rugs and cords away from anywhere I would be moving. I moved the bed away from wall so I would have plenty of room for my walker. Don't think you can't trip, go slow." Babs

"I was told to buy a grabber because I would not be able bend down. As I moved along those first days, I sometimes had to clear things out of the way, or pick up things I might have dropped. It was a help. I figured out how to attach it [the grabber] to the walker using a very small elastic cord." Ruth

Question: *What surprised you the most in the first days after surgery and how did you cope?*

"I was pretty good in remembering every detail except for my German shepherd. She's very sweet, but 85 pounds. How was I going to walk her? I had a couple of incredible neighbors who stepped right in to help." Susie Q

"I had naively expected to be able to do paperwork, etc., in bed during recovery. Not only could I not stand the weight of the laptop on my thigh, I really couldn't think clearly enough to do the work. I remember crying one day because I needed to mail a bill, and the stamps were at the other end of the house. How did I cope? By accepting I just had double knee surgery and that I wasn't super woman, that's how." Tess

"The biggest challenge for me was to sit down and rest. I am the kind of person that every time I sit down to read or knit, I remember what I forgot to do -- laundry, get the mail, feed the dog, put things away. Well, I couldn't do that. I learned patience." Emma

"I have also loved knitting, embroidery and water coloring. I have a small patio where I could sit in the sun and read. For an old lady I live an active life. Just relaxing and thinking was wonderful." Ruthie

"Be very careful. After knee surgery you can easily lose your balance and trip especially after anesthesia. My advice is to think ahead. Think about the rug in front of you or a slope in the floor or the tiles in your bathroom. Walk through your house before you have surgery and look for any problems." Susan
"Make sure someone is around or checks on you routinely, in case you fall and hurt yourself. Those first days I fell twice and thankfully my husband was there to help me get back up. I once tripped when I was getting up from the couch." Sarah

"I'll bet I'm the only one who likes to paint birdhouses. I buy the plain wooden ones at the hobby store, paint them and give them to my neighbors at Easter. That's what I did the first week. What was I going to do, play football?" Kayla

"I think other women should know that it is smart to remain still a lot of the time. I treated it like meditation and a chance to retreat inward which is funny because I wasn't that kind of person." Katherine

Common Comments: A Safe Place to Heal

There are many tricks women learned to make sure the room in which they spent most of their time was safe from tripping, falling and other hazards.

1.   Take a tour of the area before surgery. Before surgery, turn off the lights and try to get around with a scooter, walker, cane or crutch. Are you tripping or bumping into anything? Fix it!

2.   Figure out how you will get to the bathroom *with a walker*, from where you are resting, sitting or at a desk. Do this ahead of time.

3.   After surgery, and especially with needing to use a walker, it is a good idea to use night lights and to install light switches that have built in lights.

4.   Eliminate small throw rugs particularly if you have wooden floors.

5.   All cords off of the floor, not just electrical cords, but cords from blinds and curtains.

6.   Replace clock radios or alarms with your cell phone.

7.   Create a "zone" that is free of kids toys and pet toys.

8.   Slick magazines, plastic coverings, throw pillows, blankets, plant stands are all tripping hazards.

9.   Try to move furniture that are "hooking hazards," such as legs that a foot can hook around.

10.   Move glass tables or any furniture with sharp edges.

11.   If there is no one at home for you, give house keys to a friend.

12.   Is there a small leak on a slippery surface anywhere you might be walking? This can include a roof leak, condensation from a humidifier or air conditioner or even a potentially slippery area in the winter such as a porch. Please fix these things.

13.   Be VERY careful of lit candles and fireplaces. Fire is a real threat. Your new knee will slow you down.

14.   Area heaters, especially the old kinds can be dangerous if toppled. By a new one if you need to do so or borrow a safe one from a friend.

15.   If it's winter and you know the sidewalks, patio or porch can be slippery from ice, be extremely careful. Have someone put down an indoor/outdoor mat. Better yet, don't walk there!

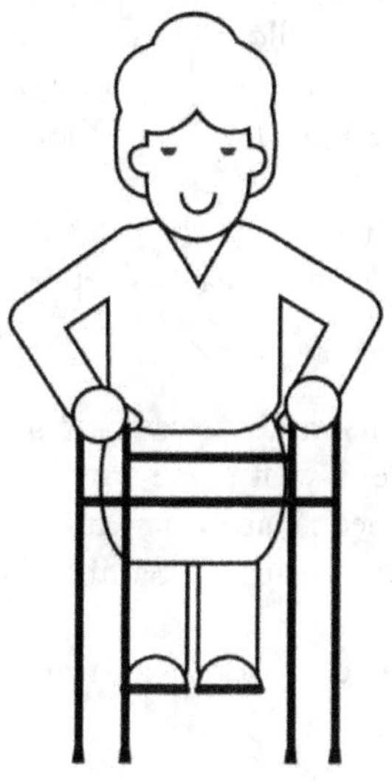

Chapter Two: Sleep, Precious Sleep

Question: *Sleeping can be a problem for women recovering from knee surgery. How did you manage?*

Sleeping is fundamental to wellness. However, as the knee begins its healing process, it may be difficult to find a comfortable sleeping position. The women we interviewed initially used three methods to get comfortable: reclining chairs, foam wedges and pillows, before being able to sleep in their usual positions. The transition "back to normal" may take days to several weeks. One thing was clear: after complete or partial knee replacement, no one was able to sleep "as usual" until time had passed. Here were some of their coping tricks:

Reclining Chairs: Using a reclining chair or a bed that could be adjusted.

"I barely slept but I'm a bad sleeper anyway. I slept on a reclining chair and used pillows under my knee. I used a sound machine to cause some white noise to help sleep in general. I also put a fan on me in case I got hot." Heather

"I slept in a recliner with an electric side control. I usually slept with my knees raised. I'm a heavy sleeper, so it wasn't an issue." Katherine

"I slept in a recliner and it was not good (comfortable). But honestly, I haven't slept well since menopause 20 years ago. For me, sleep has always been hard but with the knee it made it more difficult. I took sleep medication." Sarah

[**Note**: *Always* consult your healthcare provider in regard to medication.]

"My husband has a great recliner in our den which is his 'man cave!' but for several weeks I took over the room and that's where I slept. I elevated the knee from time to time. Sometimes I had to use a pillow. My only other problem was getting used to the Ole' Miss logo on the slip cover! I'm from Georgia!" Catherine

"I couldn't get comfortable in a bed and so I had to sleep on a recliner. I did put a pillow under my knee and that really helped." Meredith

"I used a recliner for the first few weeks, and you know what? I loved it! My surgery was in the winter and I bundled heavy quilts on top of me. It was the best part of my surgery (LOL) other than a new knee that didn't hurt." Harriet

"My husband and I are big people and so a few years ago we bought a king-sized bed that could change positions. My procedure wasn't too bad. Initially I adjusted the bed so my feet were raised. I think the first night I used a pillow. Overall, it wasn't too bad." Emilie

"Sleeping worried me because the fear of my husband bumping into me was extreme. I have an adjustable bed so I was able to elevate my feet and I usually slept with the ice machine on. This combatted swelling along with the pain." Jessica

"I have a sleep number bed with an adjustable base so I was able to raise and lower the bed to a comfortable position. I was NEVER told to put pillows under my knees while healing. Maybe if my bed didn't adjust, I would have had to." Susie Q

Wedge: Using a foam wedge and/or pillows to elevate the body in the bed or couch.

"I had bilateral knee replacements; I am normally a side sleeper so I had to sleep on my back. I slept in my bed actually. I had my husband's assistance the first few nights to get in and out and to use the bathroom. In the beginning, I sometimes slept with the wedge pillow with my feet elevated. When I could finally sleep on my side, I put a pillow between my knees." Babs

"I slept on the couch with a foam wedge under my ankle and numerous pillows under my knee. It took days before I made it to bed. Still elevated my leg for weeks after surgery using the wedge combination." Kayla

"Because I did both knees at once, I didn't have a good side to sleep on, so I had to sleep on my back for weeks which I was not used to at first! I used 2 wedges under my legs to elevate them and 2 regular pillows to support my neck and back. Later, when I could turn on my side, I tried a pillow between my knees as recommended, but could never get it arranged in a way that didn't hurt one or the other. Do people who recommend these things actually know what it's like to have knee surgery? Also, the weight of even a sheet was too much so we arranged blankets to cover my lower legs and torso, leaving my knees exposed. It took time, but I made it." Tess

Pillows: Modifying the bed by loading it up with pillows of all sorts until there is adequate support and comfort.

"YES, it affected my sleep! My sleep cycle was messed up for at least 4 months after the surgery. When I would sleep, I would have restless leg and/or cramps in the surgery leg. I always kept my leg elevated with pillows and iced it right before attempting to sleep. I slept better on the sofa than in my bed and I believe this was due to my sofa being firm and I couldn't toss around too much." Pamela

"I had to get used to sleeping on my back. I slept on the couch, on my back, with a pillow beneath my knee and ankle. It really bothered me to have the heel of my foot resting on the couch so I kept it elevated." Whitney

"Initially, I had no problem sleeping as I was so drugged out! So right after surgery I came home and propped my knee up on the reclining chair. Later that night I went to bed with lots of pillows. It was very hard to find a comfortable position. It took time." Emma

"The pain made the sleeping hard, even with the meds. I slept with a pillow under my knee and I would also periodically wake up and in the beginning put ice on it throughout the night." Susan

"It was difficult to find a position so my knee didn't hurt. I had to put a pillow under my knee. Looking back, I wish I had bought a foam wedge. They really aren't that expensive." Violet

"I love my couch. I couldn't fall asleep very well lying on my back, but I put pillows under my knee until I felt a little more comfortable." Ruthie

"I slept downstairs for a few weeks because I couldn't go upstairs. To be honest, the sleeping was awful. I slept on a big, round chair in the living room. The living room doesn't have the best curtains so it was bright and the position was not relaxing. I learned to put blankets under my legs since the pillows were not comfortable." Lori

"I need to be truthful. Sleep was miserable for me. I felt trapped not being able to move my knee for so long, along with swelling and keeping it elevated. I arranged pillows under my knee to elevate it, and pillows for my lower back as well." Michelle

Common Comments: Sleep is Good

1. Be prepared to sleep in a different position in the days or even weeks following surgery.
2. Stairs might be a problem. If you need to sleep in a different place, such as the living room or a den, make sure drapes or blinds shut out the light. If strange appliance noises bother you, consider getting one of those white-noise machines.
3. Though pets are affectionate and comforting, unless you have a Chihuahua or Pomeranian, the family St. Bernard or Golden Retriever should not be encouraged to jump on the recliner!
4. Ice packs or ice machines can be your best friends. Consult with your doctor or physical therapist before surgery about the use of ice to help you ease the pain during the night.
5. **Make sure you can *easily* reach a light or at least a flashlight, especially if you are sleeping in an unfamiliar place.**

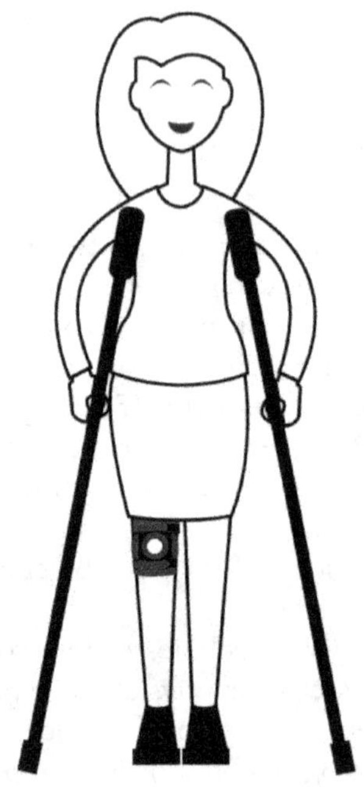

Chapter Three: Relaxation

Question: *What did you do to relax?*

"As the pain diminished, my favorite way to relax was a glass of wine and spending time in my beautiful garden. I think my garden healed me more than anything." Samantha

"Audiobooks are wonderful. There's literally anything on line. Reading in general was relaxing and knitting really helped me to get my mind off minor aches and pains." Emma

"I would do breathing exercises that I have learned in the past to help my anxiety. I had a lot of anxiety after surgery, wondering if I would ever be the same. And being cooped up in the house made it worse as well. So breathing deeply and slowly helped me with pain and anxiety." Lori

"I hated being on pain medication and so I got off it as fast as I could. I played with my kids when I could and watched a lot of movies." Anne

[**Note:** *Always* consult your healthcare provider in regard to medication.]

"I drank some wine and talked to friends. I would find exciting books to read to take my mind off of it all. I would also sit in the garden which was helpful. Being in nature is important." Michelle

"My faith is what and continues to keep me going. I would pray when I was in a lot of pain and still continue to do so." Susan

"I don't know if I already mentioned this, but I was a serious musician. I had abandoned my music but after my arthroscopy I found that playing the flute helped me to relax. I guess it's one of the nice things about being forced to relax. You get to know yourself again." Emilie

"Anything that would take my mind off discomfort. I read, I love adult coloring books, crossword puzzles, sudoku or just watching TV." Pamela

"I knitted up a storm. I made sweaters for two grandkids and baby booties for the neighbor's newborn. It helped the pain go away when I focused." Ruthie

"I sort of did meditation each night, reminding myself that while I was in a lot of pain when I was moving, I wasn't in pain while lying still…I visualized all the day's pain draining out and away, starting with my head and working downward. I do think it helped me to fall asleep." Tess

"I started to do guided meditations after knee surgery. It made me more accepting because I know my knees would never be the same. I accepted my knee would never be the same." Sarah

"I bought a language program. I got back to my Spanish. I did so well, I want to visit Panama soon. It relaxed me whenever I was in pain." Harriet

"I don't think I did much, I am more of a mind over matter person. I powered through. Gluten free diet, etc. This helps with pain but most people want to mask pain instead of change of diet to help." Heather

Common Comments: Watch Where You Walk!

Sometimes, the most treacherous times to move around, are not the times right after knee surgery, but when you're thinking, "I got this and I can power through this!" It's OK to feel optimistic, but don't get ahead of yourself. Taking those bold first steps with walkers, crutches or canes might cause you to quickly learn that hidden challenges can be found most anywhere. Though some of these "dangers" might seem obvious and almost condescending to mention, many of the women who responded felt that it was *the little dangers that could get you anytime*. Be aware of the following situations:

1. Snow and ice – Assume you'll slip and fall. Get help!
2. Floors in malls and department stores – Those "danger signs" are intended for you!
3. Grocery stores, ESPECIALLY when a customer spilled liquid
4. Shower stalls and bathtubs – BOTH are scary. Be EXTRA careful.
5. Locker rooms and all gym floors
6. Soapy floors of any kind, any surface

7.   Poolside
8.   Throw rugs on wood or linoleum
9.   Linoleum and porcelain tile
10. Gravel surfaces

Floors in "dark areas" such as movie theaters, stadiums, concert halls, restaurants and bars (Remember that alcohol consumption and knee surgery don't mix very well!)

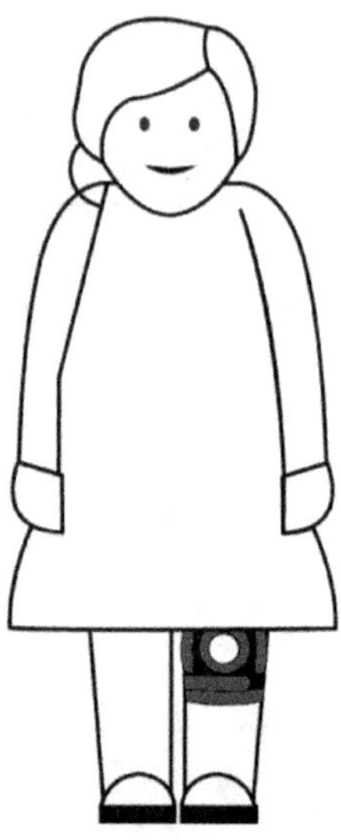

Chapter 4: Heat and Ice

Question: *Looking back did you favor heat or ice for comfort? Please explain.*

[**Note**: *Always* consult your healthcare provider in regard to treating pain.]

In general, the women we interviewed used both cold and hot to soothe pain, but cool or cold was preferred. If nothing else, there were plenty of frozen vegetables left over after the knees healed!

"When I did my first knee, I ended up buying the type of ice packs used by my physical therapist. They are large and can be strapped to your knee." Suzie Q

"I used ice going back to my sports injuries in college. Ice was like my best friend. Insurance didn't cover my ice machine and I didn't care. When you're done with your healing you can still use it for all kinds of aches and pains." Anne

"Both really. When I needed ice, I used old-fashioned ice packs and I froze small water bottles and wrapped them in a dish towel." Sarah

"Always cold. I used ice packs and my favorite, bags of frozen peas, they form around your knee a lot better." Meredith

"Ice right after, but I'm not a 'cold person.' I enjoyed hot baths in the months to follow." Harriet

"When the leg cramps and restless leg were at their worst, I used heat to relax the muscles. Both my surgeon and my physical therapist advised against heat on the surgical site for a month or longer. A recipe my physical therapist gave me was to mix rubbing alcohol and water to make a slushy ice mixture. I put it in freezer bags, stuck it in the freezer and had one ready when I needed it. You can look it up on line." Pam

"Before I went into surgery and I was in pain, we bought bags of ice several times a week because our ice maker couldn't keep up. After, I used the ice machine I got from the hospital. It stayed cold for longer periods of time." Jessica

"Heat. Heat worked well for me. I sometimes used frozen water bottles though that I wrapped in a towel." Katherine

"Both heat and ice but ice worked better. I used a bag of veggies during the day but at night I used actual ice packs." Susan
"Frozen beans worked well for me!" Whitney

"I had an ice machine for the first surgery. It was a challenge. So, I used ice packs for the second surgery and they worked fine." Violet

"I used both heat and cold intermittently, heat for like 5 minutes and then ice for 3 and so forth. I think it helped. For cold I used ice packs, the sports injury ones." Lori

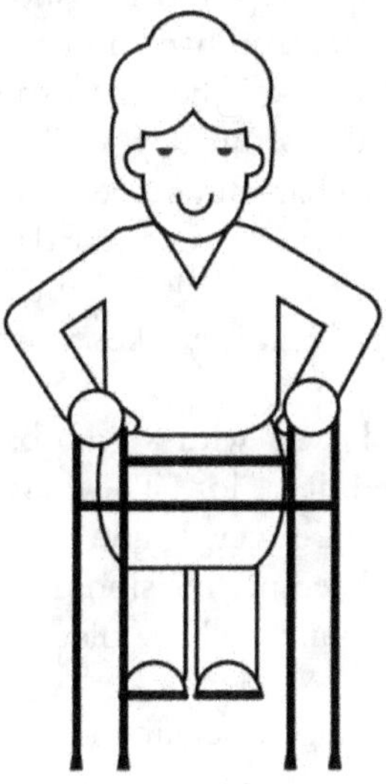

Chapter 5: Personal Hygiene

Question: *In the first weeks following surgery were there unexpected personal hygiene challenges? How did you cope with them?*

Showering

"Yes, showering was difficult at first. *It is dangerous so have help.* My spouse had to help me wash and to make sure my balance and standing were OK. In terms of keeping my incision dry, I used waterproof bandages." Kayla

"Taking a shower after the sutures were removed was troublesome. I had to step into the shower and balance myself at the same time. My husband had to help me at first. *Don't try to do it alone.* Until you get help, it's better to smell a little! I was happy we had nonslip floors. Unfortunately, we have a small shower so I was unable to have a grab bar. But something we could do was to install a hand-held shower head. After a few days, I did find a way to keep myself clean, which was to sit on the edge of the tub and give myself sponge baths. That way I kept my incision dry." Jessica

"I have a stall shower with a grab bar. *We installed* a hand-held shower and I used it a lot. They are easy to install and not expensive. It was a life-saver. I didn't use a shower chair because it was in the way. To keep my incision dry, I used 'Press 'n Seal' food wrap and it worked quite well." Violet

"Yes, I did use a shower chair and it worked best for me. In the very beginning I took sponge baths, so the shower chair worked out well. My biggest problem was wrapping my knee in plastic when I had to shower. This is why sponge baths were so great." Michelle

"*At first, my husband helped me get in the shower.* The safest thing for me to do was to do was to do as much as possible from a seated position. I did LOTS of sponge baths and I used a shower chair." Tess

"My procedure was pretty simple compared to a total replacement, but I had trouble moving around in the shower. A grab bar was already in place in the shower. One night I slipped and almost fell. I'm young but if I was older, I could have done serious damage. Get a grab bar. Please don't be stupid." Emilie

"You must have a grab bar for the tub, anyway that's my opinion. It's way too dangerous otherwise. I bought a shower transfer bench to go from outside the bathtub and to slide into the shower. They're adjustable no matter how high your bathtub. Set it up before surgery so you can get used to it beforehand." Babs

"I ordered a grab bar for safety on Amazon. I usually gave myself sponge baths at the beginning because it was safer. I used waterproof bandages on my incision and then wrapped my knee in a trash bag to be extra safe." Heather

"I used a shower chair because I was afraid of falling. At least have a bath mat." Ruthie

"I had to test things out after my operation. What I did was to wrap my knee in plastic and gave myself sponge baths. I sat on the edge of the tub and that helped with safety. I think that in the days after the operation it is better to sit than stand." Katherine

"Don't try to do a balancing act in the shower. Go on Amazon to find long-handled washing brushes and sponges. Do your back and legs that way." – Emilie

"*A friend helped me in and out of the shower at first.* Don't do it alone. If you drop something like a shampoo bottle, leave it there or have a friend retrieve it later. My shower is too small for a chair, but it could be a good idea I think." Harriet

Common Comments: Showering

1. Get help until you are absolutely steady on your own. Don't be brave, be smart.
2. If you can, install a grab bar and/or a handheld shower.
3. If the floor of the shower is normally slippery at least get a bathmat.
4. Talk to your healthcare provider as to when you no longer need to keep the incision dry.
5. Make sure all containers you use are unbreakable.
6. Soap is a major danger be cautious if anything slips from your hand. This is why help is a good idea.
7. If you like your privacy, at least keep the bathroom door unlocked in case of an accident.

The Toilet

"Sitting down and getting up were the difficult parts. We bought a small foot-stool that I could put my feet on which helped keep my knees at an OK angle. I was also able to slide my walker back over the toilet (with the front facing the tank) so I had 'chair arms' to push myself up with. In the very beginning, I was in a lot of discomfort. The absolute best gadget for me was a female urination device (Camping Travel Toilet Urination Device). It was great for peeing at night so I could pee standing up. They are available in some camping stores and on Amazon for under $15. I also took it with me to use in public restrooms where there were no tall handicapped toilets." Tess

"Using the toilet is challenging and getting up could be challenging. I found that if I kicked the surgery leg to the side, I was able to get up a little better and it was less painful." Jessica

"Getting up from the toilet was hard. My husband put a chair next to it, so I could get balanced before standing." Michelle

"I should have taken fiber supplements a few days before surgery. In the beginning, I spent a lot of time in the bathroom waiting for something to happen!" Whitney

"I bought a toilet riser with handles because it would have hurt me too much to get up and down from the normal level." Babs

"I thought that my upper body strength could help me overcome everything. Getting up from a seated position such as the toilet was hard at first. My mother-in-law gave me a raised toilet seat with handles before my surgery. I told her I didn't want any part of it, that it was for old ladies. In a million years I never thought I would use it. Guess what? I used it for almost two weeks." Anne

"Using the toilet was very hard, I needed help getting up a lot. Thankfully we have been married for a long time! My husband was there to help." Sarah

Other Hygiene Concerns and Tips

"I sat down to do most things such as my hair and make-up. However, I could not shave my legs without creating a dangerous situation and that was awful for me. Just let it go." Lori

"It was painful to stand so I used a chair for doing my hair. I'm a teacher so luckily school was out so I did not have to do my make-up daily." Pam

"When I was brushing my teeth or brushing my hair, I kept the walker in front of me because I could get off balance and I had something to grab on to in case I started to fall. Chances are your new knees will make you feel off-balance at first." Babs

"Balancing to brush the teeth and to gargle was harder than I thought." Sarah

"Because I was off-balance, doing my hair was harder than I thought it would be." Susan

Comments about Skin Care

"My skin was very itchy. I used lotion where I could a few times a day." Whitney

"My incisions on both knees itched a lot. I got the surgeries years apart, but for both knees it itched like crazy and I hated it." Heather

"Everything was itchy after surgery; I don't know why. I bought a lotion applicator for my back and when my husband wasn't around, I applied lotion to my back and legs." Emilie

"The antibiotic soap they had me use dried me out. I was able to apply lotion after the surgery but not to the surgery site." Jessica

"As a matter of fact, my skin was drier after surgery. I don't know why. I had one of my friends buy me some really good lotion." Pamela

Common Comments: Shared Personal Care Tips

1. Seated positions are safest at first.
2. In the beginning, everything will be more difficult. Before surgery try doing your hair, brushing your teeth, etc., from a seated position.
3. Using the toilet may be a problem. Several women suggested buying a raised toilet set with or without handrails.
4. Ask your healthcare provider about starting on a fiber supplement *prior to surgery*. Anesthesia has been known to cause constipation.
5. If you have the room in your shower area consider buying a "shower seat" for those first few days or weeks when you feel unsteady.
6. Expect your balance to be off. Several women recommended hairdryer holders and that way one hand can be used for balancing.
7. Before surgery, consider buying small, cheap plastic dispenser bottles and filling them with your favorite shampoo, conditioner, mouthwash and other liquids. Never bring anything made of glass into the shower.
8. They still sell spray deodorants if it's easier to balance while doing that than using a roll-on.
9. For hydration, buy a good quality water bottle. It is less clumsy than those cheap bottles of water, more economical and reduces environmental impact.
10. Because of balance issues and difficulty walking, keep a supply of hand sanitizer close by your chair instead taking of too many trips to the sink.

11. Laxatives! Whether you favor Metamucil, stool softeners, herbal laxative teas, lots of water, prune juice or something else, every woman interviewed said that due to anesthesia, it's a safe guess it will take a while before you're "regular." Talk to your physician or nurse about it beforehand.

12. Carry a phone with you, especially if you live alone and run into unexpected personal hygiene problems.

13. Consider a grab bar by the toilet in addition to one in the shower.

14. You may not need it, but ask your surgeon about keeping a small supply of extra waterproof dressings.

15. DON'T try to stand on a stool or bench to adjust the shower head.

16. Several women suggested that getting short, easy to manage hair styling was the best way to go. By the time it grows out, you will be much better!

17. Other short-cuts to hair care mentioned included no-rinse shampoos, hair turbans, scrunchies and hair straightening combs.

18. Scratching an itch while balancing on one knee? Forget it. The women recommended telescopic back-scratchers and several companies sell long-handled lotion applicators.

19. Shaving can be a problem, a few women mentioned that there are companies that make razors with shaving cream inside them easier to use while healing.

20. Travel-sized "everything" including deodorants, mouthwash, creams, shampoos and conditioners. If you're going to be on business trips before surgery keep all the hotel "samples."

21. Dental picks rather than floss or tape. You can easily use them with one hand.

22. Toothpaste comes in flip-top containers so you can't drop the cap!

23. Several women favored water flossers as an easy to use oral hygiene tool.

24. There are a few companies that make travel toothbrushes with the toothpaste built into the handle.

25. Prior to surgery, *make a list of all of the personal hygiene products you expect to use over the course of six weeks.* Have the

supply in a readily reachable place, not out in a garage or a difficult to reach shelf.

26. Finally, re-fill your prescriptions prior to surgery.

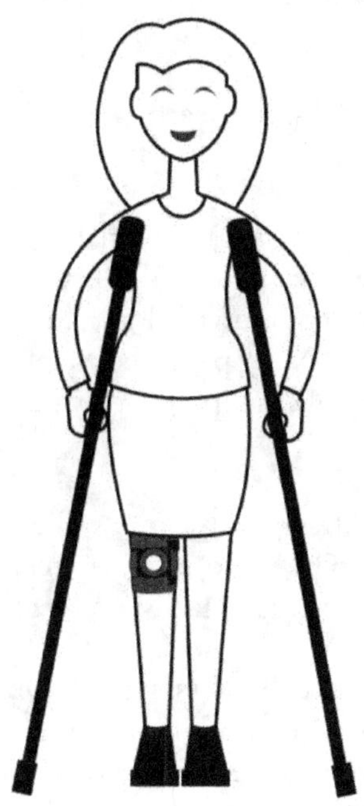

Chapter 6: The "Survival Basket"

Question: *Did you make up a "Survival Basket?" What was in it?*

Some women called them "Survival Baskets," while others called them "Knee Stations" or simply, daily "essential" supplies. After replacement surgery you're probably not going to want to walk around very much. Most women elect to be in one spot and have the necessary supplies at hand.

Sometimes a wicker or plastic basket from the dollar store fits the bill, or a small, designated table top, or more advanced, a little red wagon that you drag from room to room.

"I kept the following things on a small table near my favorite chair: bottled water, a small plastic bag filled with trail mix, iPhone charger, TV remote and lip balm." Emma

"I always had a book nearby, the TV remote and water." Samantha

"Yes, I had a basket set-up with hand lotion, dark chocolate (my favorite), pretzels, phone and charger, water and a book. My skin got very dry after surgery, I don't know why. I also made up a basket for the kitchen with paper cups, plates, napkins and plastic sporks. I didn't feel like slipping on water from washing dishes." Michelle

"I had a bag attached to my walker that I purchased on Amazon. Kept my pills, a notepad to keep track of when I took them, my cell phone, water, snacks, and a grabber." Harriet

"Actually, I had two baskets set up. One in the bathroom and one by the recliner. In the bathroom, I had toothpaste and toothbrush, hair brushes, nail file and scissors, mouthwash, razor, tampons, shave cream, skin lotion and medications. It made it easier for me.

In the other basket I always kept water, body lotion, granola, the cell phone charger and the remote. My husband left chocolate for me at first and I loved it, but I didn't want to pack on too much weight!" Anne

"I kept the console on the sectional full of anything I might need. I ALWAYS had my cell phone with me in case I ran into trouble. Some of the stuff around me were my iPad, tissues, flash light, puzzle books, the remotes, snacks and water." Jessica

"It wasn't fancy, but I tossed things in a basket like lotion, snack foods, cell phone charger, etc., but after a while I carried my backpack around rather than having a basket hanging off my walker." Tess

"I put together a large basket with my computer and phone, always water and snacks. I liked having lavender lotion and again the lavender smell was a help for my anxiety." Lori

"In addition to water, lotion and snacks, I kept my medicine near me, a few books, iPad, and a dog brush! I found it relaxing to groom our Golden retriever. By the way, I have a friend who had a full knee replacement. She lives in a small house and what she did was to take over her toddler's wagon, load it with her stuff, and take it room to room!" Emilie

"Hand sanitizer, lotion, iPad, something to drink, charger and remote. Hand sanitizer is really important I think, because my personal hygiene didn't get back to normal for about 10 days. I had a basket by my recliner. Every morning my husband would bring me a cup of coffee and a banana, so I had them when I woke up!" Meredith

"I had a lot of trouble sleeping and a lot of itching. In my basket I put in an eye mask to block out the light, even lavender oil. I also put a white noise machine near my chair. I bought some really good skin lotion, put in in the basket and used it all the time." – Suzie Q

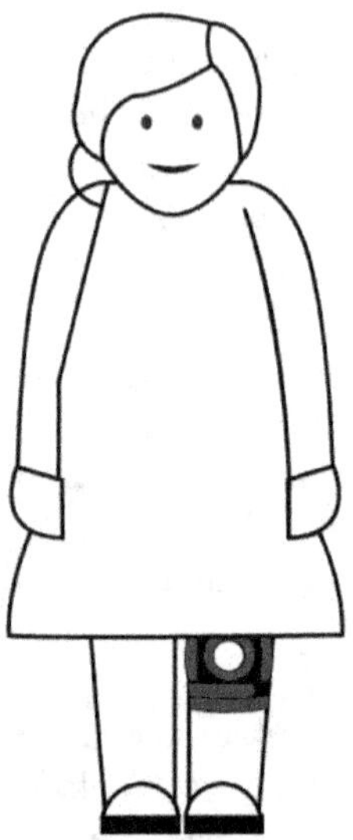

Chapter 7: The Wardrobe, Function over Style

Question: *What was your wardrobe like those first days or weeks? Did you have any trouble wearing things?*

"Right after surgery I wore sweat pants a size larger than I usually wear. My local drugstore sometimes has them for sale cheap and I hit it right, about 10 days before I went in. They were easier to pull up and down. I wanted *nothing* touching my leg so this made it less painful. The only thing I had trouble putting on were panties. I often wore a robe around the house. Get a good robe before you go into the hospital." Jessica

"The most difficult thing to put on was underwear. Lying down might be easier for you when are putting underwear on. I'll be honest, I'm an old woman and I have a lot of loose clothes. If you need something, go to Walmart and buy the cheapest clothes you can find. Don't spend a fortune." Sarah

"Nice PJs with a sweater over the top made it easy to feel dressed-enough when we had visitors. This was not the time to impress anyone. They should have been happy enough to know I ran a brush through my hair! I kept wearing my hospital issued, no-slip socks. Later on, I wore loose, long-elastic waist skirts and socks. By the way, I didn't wear regular jeans for months then finally jeans when my skin was not so sensitive to the rough fabric." Tess

"Underwear was the toughest things to put on and once I got that on, I spent my days in shorts and T-shirts. I could not stand any kind of tight clothes on me." Kayla

"I had surgery in the middle of winter. My uniform was a robe over a nightgown and wool socks. I graduated to wearing lots of leggings. I would recommend to women to buy leggings or wide loose pants and sweaters." Emma

"I practically lived in baggy sweat pants and a sweat shirt and old lady underwear! Sometimes, simple dresses. They are awesome after surgery. I'm a huge fan of jeans, but forget about it on top of an incision. The lightest clothing feels like it weighs a ton." Meredith

"I'm a big fan of Walmart, Target or Goodwill. Before my surgery I went to Goodwill and bought a couple huge sweatshirts and sweatpants, washed the "H" out of them and they served me well. Funny story. One sweatshirt said 'Harvard Medical School.' An acquaintance of a friend asked if I went there. 'Sure,' I said, 'Right after I graduated from plumbing school.'" Harriet

"I hated putting on socks. I know there's a gadget they sell where you stretch the socks and then put them on by pulling on a cord. I never got the hang of it. I usually dressed in stretchy pants and a loose top. To put on pants, I held onto a railing for balance and kind of stepped into them and pulled them up. I suppose if you have knee replacement surgery in the winter you could put on a fuzzy sweater over the top." Violet

"I wore comfortable workout shorts at first. I recommend that you wear things that are elastic in the waist as they are easy to put on and take off. Loose clothing is critical. Shorts are helpful as you can monitor the knee. Before surgery I bought a few cheap dresses and shorts from Target. Underwear is the hardest thing to put on because it's hard to stretch and balance. Practice before surgery! You may have to steady yourself when putting on shorts and underwear." Michelle

"Go to the thrift store and buy oversized men's shirts and if you're nervous about bedbugs (ha-ha) get them laundered the first time around. They look fine with shorts too. Also, I bought 'kimono sleeve' tunics on Amazon. In the first weeks that's as dressy as I could get." Emilie

"I recommend comfy clothes, sweats and loose shirts. Make sure and have pants or shorts that are super loose so they can get over your knee. The biggest problem I had was putting on socks. I couldn't bend that far or reach that far. I needed help." Katherine

"I found what they called 'kimono loose-fit tunics.' I didn't feel like standing around and getting dressed. They are stretchy enough to put on and to take off in almost any position. They look nice with a skirt, baggy sweatpants or loose-fitting pants. Don't spend a lot of money on clothes. You're not going to want to do much, you just want to look half-human for your mother-in-law!" Anne

"Things that are comfortable are the most important! Don't care about how you look, try to be comfortable. I lived in loose shorts, and when we were able to go out, I wore a skirt. You will probably have trouble putting on underwear at first. I often put on clothes while laying down." Susan

"I have had 3 knee replacements [one surgery was unsuccessful ha-ha!] so I guess I'm an expert on this. Find comfortable, loose-fitting bottoms. You'll need to be able to do exercises in whatever you're wearing and what you look like isn't your priority here. You need to be able to work that knee/leg freely. I ran into an issue with my left knee, where I could hardly stand the touch of fabric against my skin due to the highly sensitized nerve endings along the incision. Fortunately, that surgery was in July so I could sleep with my leg uncovered and wear shorts during the day. When I went back to work in the early fall, I was able to wear lightweight skirts but as the weather got cooler, I had to go to lightweight slacks." Suzie Q

"Loose shorts are the only way to go. Underwear is miserable to put on! I dressed like I was going to the gym except for the sneakers part." Whitney

"I wore dresses, real loose pants. In fact, here's the rule to everyone: Loose, loose and looser. I already had cheap, bulky sweaters and sweatshirts I bought at Walmart. At home, I am a cozy person so I liked that kind of stuff already." Lori

"Don't care about looking good or stylish. Pajama pants helped me but also comfortable shorts. Almost everything I tried to put on was uncomfortable. It's kind of like a game and when the pain goes away and you can walk, you won!" Heather

Common Comments: Clothing

1. Panties are the most difficult article of clothing to put on; try practicing before surgery by lying flat on your back and cinching them up that way.
2. Socks can be difficult. They make "sock-grabbers" that some women master and others don't. See if a friend might have a sock-grabber and determine if you could use it.
3. Many women reported that *any weight* on the incision was uncomfortable. Lightweight or very loose sweatpants, skirts or tunics may be a better solution.
4. Go for comfort, not fashion.

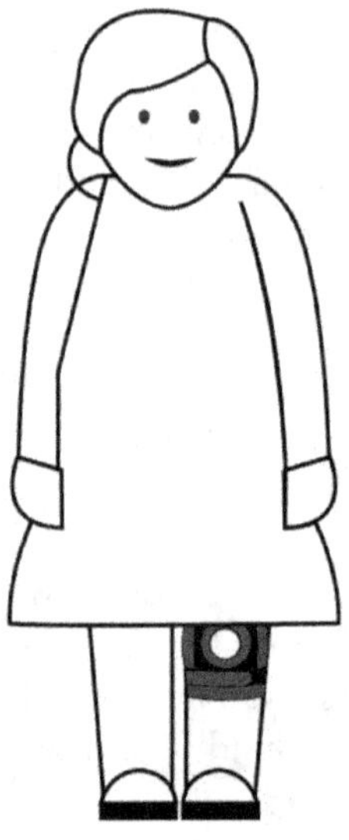

Chapter 7: Footwear &Etc.

Question:*In the first few weeks, what was your footwear of choice?*

"I wore sandals that I could slip on. If I went out, I wore slip-on shoes that had no laces. I could not wear socks for a while, and NO to hose!" Michelle

"I liked slip-on shoes, no laces. You can find lots on Amazon. I could wear socks but they were hard to put on." Violet

"At first, I lived in my flip-flops, but one day, I almost tripped and fell. After that, I switched to clogs. They were also better in the kitchen and provided a little more support." Anne

"I wore slip on canvas shoes except for physical therapy. I wore tennis shoes to physical therapy, and my husband helped me at first with putting on shoes and tying laces. I always wore socks and to be honest, I never wear hose." Babs

"No way I could even think of hose and even in the beginning socks were hard. I gave up on them at first. I mainly wore slip on shoes with no laces." Samantha

"I usually wear low cut socks but at first it was hard for me to put them on unless I had help. I like to wear athletic shoes, pretty much on a daily basis. Right after surgery it was difficult to put shoes on or off because of my arthritis. I tied my shoes first and then slipped them on and off. I never wear hose." Pamela

"I could not bend down, so slip-on sneakers were best for me. Socks and underwear were difficult for me." Emma

"I work in a more formal business setting so on a lot of days I used to wear hose and heels. Forget about that after surgery! It was months before I felt comfortable in hose. I wore flats and on casual days I pre-tied my sneakers. I bought funny socks with animals and Disney characters. My socks became a topic of conversation." Emilie

"Ladies, forget about hose and maybe even socks at first. I wore fuzzy slippers and then, slip-on shoes." Sarah

"They make slip on shoes where the heel part flips back into place. No shoehorn required. They are stylish, considering." Harriet

"I only wore socks when I wore my tennis shoes. I was unable to bend when I had to tie them, so I had to have some help. I did not wear hose." Jessica

"Shoes and socks were the hardest things of all to put on. I lived in sandals. Because bending is hard at first, I recommend getting a 'pedi' before surgery, at least you'll look good!" Meredith

"I am in good shape, I practice yoga, but socks were the hardest thing to put on. I couldn't bend that far or reach if I was sitting or lying down. Recovering from knee surgery is a process. No hose or even yoga pants for me at first. I wore slippers for a while, then slip-on shoes before going back to normal." Katherine

"I prefer to wear clog or mule style shoes in the cold months or sandals in the summer so tying wasn't as much of an issue. If I did wear athletic shoes after a while, it was suggested to replace the shoe laces with 'curly laces,' which turns athletic shoes into slip-ons (with the assistance of a long-handled shoe horn). Yes, I could wear socks, but I needed to use a sock donner to put them on. They are easy to find online or in drug stores. I didn't wear hose until months and months later." Susie

Common Comments: Footwear

1. Flips-flops are attractive in their ease of use, but can be dangerous and unstable.
2. Bedroom slippers with smooth soles can be risky on shiny floors or wet surfaces.
3. Several sock manufacturers make socks with non-skid bottoms that are far safer than conventional socks.
4. Shoe laces can be substituted with curly laces.
5. Some women found it easier to pre-tie their shoes and then slip them on.
6. Several companies are marketing shoes with flexible heels that allow the foot to slip in, and then allow the heel to flip back into place.

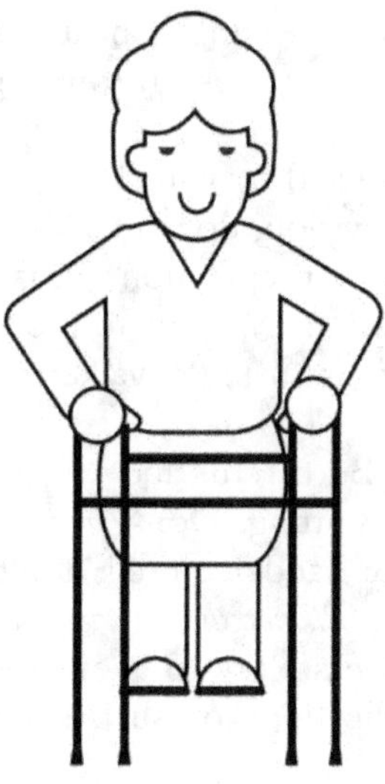

Chapter 8: Cooking Notes

Despite your absolute belief in your kitchen skills or how strong you may feel before knee surgery, *after surgery* it will be a while before you have your legs under you. *Accidents can and do happen.* Your balance will be off and it is guaranteed that your ability to move around the kitchen may be hampered.

We have compiled the top 7 safety high points that appear on almost every cooking safety list. We found it important to discuss these rules before you returned from the hospital with your repaired knee (remember, when all else fails, 'take-out' works too!).

1. **FIRE!** Got your attention? Watch yourself around the stove whether gas, electric or — if you should decide to try it — BBQ. And speaking of heat, always use potholders.
2. Please take up any loose throw rugs that may be in the kitchen.
3. Don't be distracted by your kids, company, text messages, music, the television, dogs or cats, and don't try to speed through the food preparation. Please, *focus on the kitchen task at hand.* You will not be able to move around as normal for a while. If you are using a walker or crutches be especially mindful.
4. Knife safety. Be careful and watch how you are holding the knife and cutting. Don't get off balance. If the knife slips from your hand, let it fall; don't try to grab it.
5. *Wear shoes that will not slip on the kitchen floor.* This might be hard to do at first. Try to avoid food preparation in bare feet, socks, flip-flops or slick slippers. Please, get some help.
6. *Anything spilled needs to be immediately cleaned up,* especially oils, ice water and small grains such as rice and barley. Obviously, you will have trouble doing this at first. Please, get some help.
7. *Do NOT lift anything that is too heavy for you,* a full soup pot to a heavy-duty mixing appliance can be potentially dangerous. Wait for help if something is too heavy.
8. If you have purchased a new kitchen utensil or piece of equipment, *get familiar with it before your surgery,* or have someone watch you use it after surgery. We know this might sound strange, but think about using any appliance or utensil while you are recovering and may be unsteady.
9. Boiling liquids such as soups, stews and even water for pasta are dangerous for those who are down to hobbling on one "good knee" or when using a walker. Spilled boiling water can potentially result in second degree burns. Wait for help.

Interesting Kitchen gadgets you may not know about

Over time, orthopedic surgery recovery patients have been kind enough to share all kinds of gadgetry that made life simpler for them in the kitchen in the weeks following surgery. Remember that you may be off-balance at first. The easier you can make meal preparation, the better – that's what these gadgets can do!

1. Adjustable kitchen stool – Many women recovering from knee surgery found that an adjustable stool at counter height made it easier for them to work from a seated position than by standing and trying to reach over a walker.
2. Battery operated pepper mills – These can also be used for sea salt.
3. Hand blenders – They're much easier to use than a full-size mixer.
4. Paring boards – Sometimes they're also called "Swedish cutting boards." They're very clever. They let you cut things with one hand and you can change the positions of the pins to accommodate what you want to cut.
5. Miniature food processors – They make miniature food processors and blenders that can be handled with one hand.
6. Citrus sectioning tools – One-handed tools to help you cut large oranges and grapefruits into sections.
7. "Solo Grip" – One-handed jar opener. It's plastic and you jam the jar into it and can twist off the screw-top cap with one hand.
8. Saucepan Stirrer – Come in several variations, either over the pot or in the pot, but the best news is that they are hands-free.
9. Jar-lid popper – Very clever gadget to pop the top of a glass jar one-handed.
10. Banana and apple slicers - These are fun and make fruit salads easier to prepare.

General Cooking Comments

The knee surgery recovery patients shared general cooking tips and food preparation ideas that may be useful. Orthopedic surgery "changes the equation" at first. Even if some of these suggestions seem silly, think about them and if they could potentially help you.

"Prior to surgery I should have prepared many meals and froze them. I didn't. One thing I did right in my opinion is that I moved several pots and cutting boards to the counter from the cabinets under the counter and I brought the food processor in from the garage. This way I could do everything on one level but it was still hard. I think someone should have told me that knee surgery would heighten my anxiety about doing things like cooking. I would have prepared more for that." Lori

"When I was first hobbling around, I didn't feel like cooking anything, I'm a big fan of Uber Eats, but there's plenty of services like Grub Hub you can use to deliver food to you." Whitney

"I didn't try cooking after my knee replacements. Balancing in front of the stove while using a walker was scary for me, especially as I have a gas stove. I ate a lot of things that didn't require cooking. The good news is that I often filled up on a lot of celery sticks and carrots and I wound up losing a little weight! Most of my life is based on a holistic approach to health. I ate as healthy as I could." Heather

"I did pre-prepare many things. I need to say to women 'Clear your schedule for 6 weeks.' No really, I mean it (I thought I'd be able to do many things. I couldn't). It includes cooking like normal. My church started a 'Meal Train' on-line app where people can sign up and bring meals. It was absolutely invaluable! I couldn't really cook, my husband was working and looking after me and it was great to have food arrive. And, as important as the food, was having people stop by just to check in and it helped me not feel so isolated and alone. Of course, now I am paying it forward." Tess

"My husband travels a lot and in the first couple of weeks, several friends came by the house to drop off food. My knees hurt a lot and I didn't feel like standing and cooking." Emma

"I should have prepared a lot of dishes like stews and casseroles and I didn't. It was a big mistake." Meredith

"I pre-prepared and froze a week's worth of dinners before my surgery and then several friends pitched in to help." Michelle

"Yes, I pre-prepared several meals. My husband cannot cook to save his life." Samantha

"There are some decent frozen meals on the market now and we stocked up on some before my surgery. When my husband was away on business, I made a few and they weren't that bad. Just watch the sodium in some of them." Anne

"I made several crockpot meals and froze them. I did not feel like spending time in the kitchen after surgery. I was warned about this by another knee replacement patients." Sarah

"I was not prepared for how my energy level would diminish in the beginning. Ladies from my church prepared meals and brought them over. I am very thankful." Pamela

"I like salads and energy bars. Those were my main snacks during the day while I was still recovering. I drank a lot of water because the energy bars can clog you up." Emilie

"In my experience you will not feel like cooking anything elaborate at first. I bought unit portions of foods such as frozen, crusted cod. I froze meals for a couple of weeks' worth of dinners. Takeout meals were always a fun treat." Harriet

Common Comments: Food Preparation

1. Pre-prepared meals seem the way to go.
2. Social clubs and houses of worship frequently have committees organized to deliver food to the infirm.
3. Forget about preparing elaborate meals after surgery; you'll be tired and due to being unsteady, it can be dangerous.
4. Make things easy; put appliances and pots on the counter along with plates and utensils. Don't bend down or reach up too much. "Waist-high" is plenty good enough.

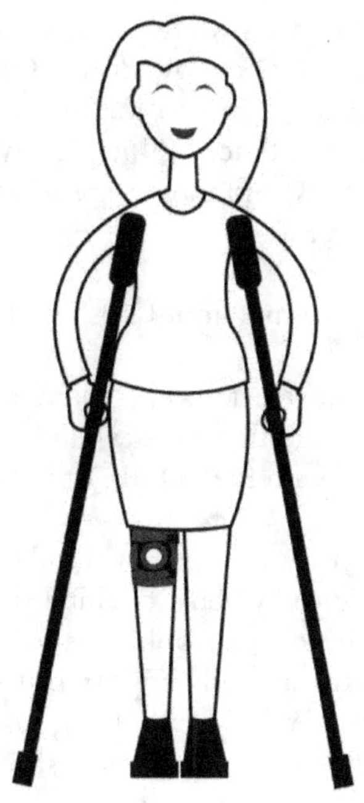

Chapter 9: "Fright Night"

Question:*Did anything frighten you at the beginning?*

"I did most of my recovery downstairs, but after I moved up to the bedroom, I became afraid of going down stairs." Lori

"I was always afraid of slipping on one of the kid's toys. You know that show *Bridezilla*? I became Mommy-zilla. I was always telling them to keep their toys away. Of course, they're young, so my husband took over those duties. At least it kept the floors clean!" Anne

"Getting up in the middle of the night to use the bathroom and whenever I had to use the stairs scared me a lot." Babs

"I did my surgery in the winter and I was afraid to slip on the ice or snow. It taught me to slow down. One thing we did was to buy an electrically heated pad to put out in front of the door to melt away the snow and ice. [Note: They are called residential snow-melting stair mats, and they come in various sizes.] I was also afraid of stairs." Emma

"Stairs were hard for me until I got my strength back." Violet

"Going up and down stairs was hard for me. I was afraid of falling after I fell for the first time while learning to balance. After that, someone stayed with me until I got it back." Kayla

"I wasn't frightened of tasks, but mindful. I had to think things out. I was really annoyed when I couldn't do something! At first, it was almost a fun challenge, 'Look, I watered our plants! I did the laundry by myself!' It was really important for me to see even a tiny bit of progress every day. If I can share, one good thing I did was to write down each positive step: first shower alone, first cutting toenails myself, etc. It helped to be able to go back and see progress, especially on days when I was really down about it all." Tess

"I initially hurt my knee by falling down stairs, so those scared me. After surgery I was very afraid of stairs for months. Be sure you have a railing." Meredith

"Cooking was very hard for me. I was off balance and it hurt to stand. I was afraid of slipping. Sometimes the best solution was food delivery." Susan

"Cleaning up or showering were rough. You have to remember to move very slowly and also, cleaning floors and shower can be dangerous." Michelle

"I was scared of falling a lot, cooking was hard, and any cleaning was hard as well. I love a clean house, but I had to let some of that go while healing." Samantha

"I had dreams about driving while my knees were bandaged and weak. I crashed or was veering off the road. It was more than enough to make me stay away from my car until I was fully healed." Ruthie

"To be honest, walking made me frightened, even to the mailbox or in the grocery store. I tried not to be alone when I first started walking. I NEVER walked with the dog." Pamela

"My procedure was no big deal. Still, thinking back, I was afraid of going down stairs at first and also, call me crazy, I was afraid of the power going out where I could not find my way at night." Harriet

"Stairs and cold. I did not go out often and the cold made it worse. We have an attached garage which made a big difference getting in and out of the car. Walking on the street with crutches was stressful because I was terrified of slipping on the ice. I did not go out much." Sarah

"Going down stairs was difficult, and also slipping on snow or ice was a worry. I had my surgery towards the end of winter. I was very careful and had someone hold my hand." Katherine

Common Comments: Fears

1. Stairs appeared to be the biggest fear with new or reconstructed knees. If you are unsure or unsteady, get assistance.
2. Fears of falling and walking on their own caused panic. Ask for help – always. If you are fearful, don't be brave, be smart.
3. Snow, ice, slippery surfaces or tripping over objects (such as toys) are worries repeated over and over again and for good reason. Each fear has a solution from snow melting mats to vigilance.

4. Please…don't think of driving anything with a motor (including a golf cart) until your physical therapist and/or surgeon says you can do so.

5. Women reported that instead of worrying about the "big picture," praise yourself for even the smallest victories. A little self-praise makes every day of your recovery better!

Finally, good healing to you! You can do this!